Am I at Risk?

Also by Sheldon Cohen

Brainstorm

Possessed

The Assist

Physics and War

Hodge Podge

Bad Blood

Payback

The Assimilated

The Patient's Guide to the Complete Medical Examination and the
Prevention of Medical Errors

Am I at Risk?

The Patient's Guide to Health Risk Factors

SHELDON COHEN M.D. F.A.C.P.

iUniverse, Inc.
New York Lincoln Shanghai

Am I at Risk?
The Patient's Guide to Health Risk Factors

iUniverse books may be ordered through booksellers or by contacting:

iUniverse
2021 Pine Lake Road, Suite 100
Lincoln, NE 68512
www.iuniverse.com
1-800-Authors (1-800-288-4677)

Because of the dynamic nature of the Internet, any Web addresses or links contained in this book may have changed since publication and may no longer be valid.

The information, ideas, and suggestions in this book are not intended as a substitute for professional medical advice. Before following any suggestions contained in this book, you should consult your personal physician. Neither the author nor the publisher shall be liable or responsible for any loss or damage allegedly arising as a consequence of your use or application of any information or suggestions in this book.

ISBN: 978-0-595-46739-6 (pbk)
ISBN: 978-0-595-70469-9 (cloth)
ISBN: 978-0-595-91034-2 (ebk)

Printed in the United States of America

To the Alexian Brothers and their world-wide health care ministry

They taught me much

CONTENTS

CHAPTER 1

INTRODUCTION

Take calculated risks. That is quite different from being rash.

General George S. Patten

1885–1945

You are at risk of losing money if you purchase a stock, bet on a horse, or sit down at a poker table. The risk to your financial health can be great if you bet more than you can afford; it can be minimal if you decide to bet two dollars when your net worth is over a million.

When it comes to your life, risk is different. More often than not, your well-being is at stake. And since you have only one life to live—why gamble with risks to your health?

But many people do gamble, either because they don't know what the risks are, or, knowing them, they just don't care; they adopt a fatalistic approach. They are proud of saying, "When your number's up, it's up."

Both categories of patients should read this book: the former, because it is important to know how to prevent a serious acute or chronic illness; and the latter, because it's time to wake up and change your attitude—especially since paying attention to health risk factors could save your life.

A risk factor is something that may increase your chance of developing an illness. The something refers to how you live your life, your ancestor's genes, what you might do, what you might not do, your age, your sex, your exposure to certain products, your eating habits, how much you exercise—or do not, your size and weight, whether you smoke or not, etcetera. There are many more.

You will come up with the probability of developing an illness if you put risk factors together. The laws of probability are amazingly precise. They allow us to have lotteries and even though the chance of buying the winning ticket may be one in many millions, if enough people buy a ticket there will always be a winner. That is a guarantee.

In the same way, if one has one risk factor for an illness there is less probability of acquiring it than if one has multiple risk factors. This is true for the most part, unless the one risk factor is overwhelmingly important—smoking, for instance.

So, with this in mind, we will discuss risk factors for the most common illnesses that may end our lives, or will cause a state of chronic disability.

There are some risk factors that you have no control over, but there are others that you have complete control over. So if you have a number of the controllable risk factors, then you need to be certain that those risk factors are controlled to the greatest extent possible.

Are there any guarantees? No, but you can increase the odds that you will not become a victim, just as betting on more horses will increase the odds that you will pick the winning horse.

Remember, by analyzing your risk factors you are practicing early detection and prevention.

That is the name of the game.

So we will list those illnesses that you will have the greatest chance of acquiring during your life time, and we will take them one at a time and discuss the risk factors for each one and what you need to do to minimize your risk.

The illnesses are as follows:

1. Disease of the heart (heart attack)

2. Cancer (most common: lung, breast, ovary, prostate, colon, skin, pancreas)

3. Stroke (cerebrovascular disease)

4. Chronic lower respiratory disease (emphysema, chronic bronchitis)

5. Unintentional injuries (accidents)

6. Diabetes mellitus

7.   Influenza (flu) and Pneumonia

8.   Alzheimer's disease

9.   Kidney disease (nephritis and nephrosis)

10. Septicemia (severe infection)

11. Intentional self harm (suicide)

12. Liver disease (chronic hepatitis, cirrhosis)

13. Essential hypertension (high blood pressure)

14. Osteoporosis

15. Depression

16. Anxiety

The first three on this list (heart-cancer-stroke) constitutes about sixty percent of the causes of death in this country.

All of us should have a risk factor analysis. Besides telling us what we are at risk for, it is extremely educational, as the risk factors and the illnesses are closely identified. This is in sharp contrast to the usual medical history that mentions some risk factors but does not make the connection between the risk factor and the illness.

So let's learn about specific risks. At the completion of each discussion, you are invited to take a quiz to determine whether you have some of the risk factors for a specific illness. When you finish, take the results to your physician. You can be a great help to him or her. You are being encouraged to be proactive.

Busy physicians need your help!

The format of this book will be as follows:

I will first discuss some generalities about the illness.

I will tell you the risk factors for the illness in question.

A set of risk factor questions for each illness will follow the above.

Again, I invite you to answer these questions and learn about your vulnerabilities.

CHAPTER 2

DISEASES OF THE HEART (HEART ATTACK)

Although there are many diseases of the heart, we will limit our discussion to heart attack—the leading cause of death in the United States.

A heart attack is caused by hardening of the heart arteries, or coronary atherosclerosis.

Coronary refers to the coronary arteries, and the word atherosclerosis is of Greek origin: athero meaning pasty gruel, and sclerosis meaning hardness. So atherosclerosis is a process where fatty material, cholesterol, calcium, various cellular waste materials and other products slowly build up in the arteries inner lining forming a substance called plaque.

A sudden rupture of this plaque can cause the artery to completely obstruct resulting in the disruption of the blood flow to a portion of the heart muscle, which if large enough will cause death.

What this means is that the first symptom of coronary atherosclerosis may be quick death, so you must pay attention to the risk factors that can lead to this sudden, unexpected end.

Diseases of the heart risk factors

High blood pressure (hypertension)

As your heart pumps blood to your body, the degree to which it pumps depends upon the amount of resistance to blood flow in your arteries. The work load of your heart becomes greater as the resistance to the flow of blood increases. This puts a strain on your heart.

In addition, the effect of high blood pressure is to accelerate the process of atherosclerosis.

The risk for high blood pressure increases as you age and is also increased if you are overweight, or eat a diet too high in salt, or live a sedentary existence.

Blood pressure that can not be controlled by life-style changes (weight loss, low salt diet, exercise, stress reduction) demands anti-hypertensive medications. Failure to control high blood pressure by life style changes and medication demands a careful search for rare and unusual causes such as adrenal gland tumors or a blocked kidney artery.

Cigarette smoke (or any tobacco)

There are 4000 known chemicals in cigarette smoke and many of them are cancer producing agents, but cigarettes cause more heart attacks than they cause lung cancer and emphysema.

In the year 2000, worldwide there were 1,690,000 heart attacks among smokers. Contrast this statistic with the 850,000 lung cancer deaths due to smoking.

Tobacco smoke (first and second hand) is well known to cause damage to the inner lining of arteries by facilitating the process of atherosclerosis and promoting blood clots. This is an arterial "double whammy." No wonder cigarettes are so potent in promoting heart attacks.

The effect, of course, is the same for all of your arteries, not just your heart. So, if you smoke, do all you can to stop. Seek help if you can't. Your life may be at stake.

High blood cholesterol

Cholesterol is an important part of the artery deposits that form plaque and narrow your arteries.

Cholesterol can not dissolve in blood, so it combines with protein and then becomes soluble. This combination is called lipoprotein.

A high level of low-density lipoprotein (LDL) in your blood increases your risk for a heart attack, as LDL, or "bad" cholesterol forms part of the plaque. The level should be under 100, or as low as seventy if you have other risk factors.

High density lipoprotein level (HDL), or "good" cholesterol helps remove cholesterol from arteries. The level should be higher than forty, but the higher the better.

Total cholesterol level equals LDL plus HDL plus one-fifth of the triglyceride (see below—this formula is only valid if the triglyceride is less than 400). The total cholesterol should be less than 200. A cholesterol/HDL cholesterol ratio has been used as a risk factor for heart attack. A ratio of less than four is considered a low risk. The risk rises with an increasing ratio.

Knowing these levels of cholesterol in your blood is critically important. If the levels put you at risk, then corrective measures, including diet, exercise and possibly medication must be started.

Triglyceride

Triglycerides are derived from ingested fats, or are made in the body from carbohydrates. They are stored in your fat cells and are made available for energy requirements.

An elevated triglyceride (normal 150 or less)) is another of the many risk factors for atherosclerosis, especially when associated with the so-called metabolic syndrome (pot belly, high blood pressure, low HDL cholesterol, diabetes, or a pre-diabetic state). This is why your physician may be interested in your abdominal measurement.

You are considered at risk if you are a man with an abdominal girth greater than 40 inches, or are a woman with an abdominal girth greater than 35 inches.

Why is this? To understand the reason you need to know that most of your fat is under your skin (subcutaneous fat), but of most concern is the fat that lies in your abdominal cavity called visceral fat—the fat that lies within your omentum, a cover of tissue that hangs down from the intestine and surrounds the organs within your abdomen.

Ordinarily you should not have more than ten percent of visceral fat, but if you have a pot belly, you may have twenty-five percent or more of visceral fat. The bad news is that there is a distinct correlation between visceral fat and diabetes and heart disease. So, it behooves you to rid yourself of your pot! And researchers have learned that if you eat the proper foods (much less saturated fats replaced by polyunsaturated fats), and get appropriate exercise (one half hour per day), you will lose your visceral fat.

This message is important regardless of your age, but is increasingly critical as you age, since the older you are the greater your risk for heart disease.

Exercise programs are also important for heart health, but should be started only with your physician's approval.

So, if your triglyceride is elevated you will need to get serious about lifestyle changes:

If overweight, strive for ideal body weight by calorie reduction—reduce carbohydrates, fats and proteins.

Stop or greatly reduce your intake of alcohol, since alcohol raises triglyceride levels.

Eliminate trans fat. They promote hardening of the arteries.

Reduce saturated fat and cholesterol in your diet. They do the same.

Exercise for at least thirty minutes every day or as much as you can if approved by your physician.

Substituting carbohydrates for fat may elevate triglycerides in some people.

Salmon, sardines, mackerel, lake trout and tuna are rich in Omega-3 fatty acids, which may reduce triglyceride levels. So eat more fish and eat less red meat.

Diabetes mellitus

Diabetes is not a single disease. There are three major types:

Type 1 diabetes (insulin-dependant, also known as juvenile diabetes) is an autoimmune disease. Your immune system, instead of protecting you, destroys the insulin-producing beta cells in the pancreas. What triggers this is uncertain. Of all diabetics, ten to fifteen percent have this form. It can appear at any age, most commonly under forty. It is known as insulin dependant diabetes, because to stay alive daily insulin injections are required.

Type 2 diabetes, formerly known as non-insulin dependant diabetes, affects eighty-five to ninety percent of diabetics. This form of diabetes, striking later in life, is characterized by insulin resistance and relative insulin deficiency. Diet, oral medication and occasionally insulin injections are required for therapy. The disease is genetic in origin, but its development may be accentuated by overweight, inactivity, poor diet and high blood pressure.

Gestational diabetes mellitus (GDM) is diagnosed during pregnancy in about seven percent of pregnant women. It disappears after birth, but indicates that the mother is prone to developing type 2 diabetes and the baby is at risk for obesity and diabetes later in life.

Diabetes is a risk factor for heart disease because, if poorly controlled, the atherosclerotic process is accelerated and cholesterol levels will rise.

Lack of exercise

Inactivity leads to weight gain, which can promote type 2 diabetes. The lack of activity plus the resulting overweight strains your heart by forcing it to pump more blood to an enlarged body. Regular physical activity can reduce the risk for heart and blood vessel disease, and can also help lower blood pressure.

Obesity

Overweight may result in diabetes. The more fatty tissue you have the more your cells become resistant to insulin. Obesity leads to inactivity with all its adverse consequences.

Stress

Intermittent stress can motivate, but when the sources are multiple and prolonged, stress can be a hazard to your health.

When you lose control of the stressful events in your life, adrenalin is released; your body develops a state of readiness to react to danger—your pupils dilate, your heart beats faster, your blood pressure rises, your breathing rate increases. You are ready for flight or fight. But you can't flee and fighting would, in most instances, be undesirable, so you become irritable, angry and anxious, all signs suggesting you may be putting yourself at increased risk for heart disease.

So, it becomes important to cope: eliminate or reduce caffeine; exercise; eat balanced meals; learn how to meditate. Stress control is important. Get professional help if necessary.

Alcohol

Alcohol, in moderation (an average of one drink a day for women and two drinks a day for men), can have beneficial cardiac effects.

It increases HDL cholesterol and can inhibit clot formation. However, in excess, it enhances clot formation, can raise blood pressure, elevate triglyceride levels and promote visceral obesity—all cardiac risk factors.

Now, knowing all this, it is not recommended that you start drinking if you haven't been, or if you have been, you start drinking more.

Family history

If your grandparents, parents, or siblings have had heart attacks, you may be at risk. Your family may have inherited a genetic condition that raises "bad" cholesterol and lowers "good" cholesterol.

High blood pressure also runs in families.

Smoking and/or exposure to second hand smoke as you grew up may play a role, as can poor family eating habits (high fat diets).

If your mother or grandmother or sister had heart trouble or a heart attack before age sixty-five, or your father or grandfather or brother had heart trouble or a heart attack before aged fifty-five, you are at greater risk.

Homocysteine

Homocysteine is an amino acid that has been implicated in the promotion of atherosclerosis by damaging the inner lining of arteries and promoting clot formation.

An elevated level has been postulated as increasing one's risk for heart attack, as well as other vascular disease.

Folic acid and vitamins B-6 and B-12 break down homocysteine in the body, and, indeed, it has been shown that reduced blood levels of folic acid have been correlated with increased risk for heart attack and stroke.

Research is still being done on this correlation, so the American Heart Association has not yet called an elevated homocysteine level a cardiac risk factor, but they do endorse determining the level in those patients with a strong family history of heart disease.

If, in these patients, homocysteine is elevated, a diet high in fruits and green leafy vegetables should be consumed daily, and perhaps a multivitamin with folic acid and the B vitamins should also be taken.

C-reactive protein (CRP)

CRP is a protein found in the blood that is a marker for inflammation. In other words, an elevated CRP suggests that there is inflammation somewhere in the body. It is a non-specific test—something's wrong someplace. It is important because inflammation has been shown to play a role in the initiation and progression of atherosclerosis and cardiac disease.

Specifically, a variation of the CRP known as highly sensitive CRP, or hs-CRP has been used to predict cardiac disease. If your hs-CRP is elevated, then you should go all out on risk factor prevention and your physician may choose to treat you with anti-clot medications such as aspirin or clopidogrel and may also consider the use of statin drugs and ace inhibitors to reduce the CRP.

In a clinical trial involving 18,000 physicians, an elevated CRP was associated with a three fold increase in heart attacks.

It has also been shown that an elevated hs-CRP applies also to an increased risk for stroke and peripheral vascular disease and the likelihood of closure of a coronary artery after angioplasty.

There are also some newer inflammatory biological markers whose worth is currently being evaluated.

Fibrinogen

Fibrinogen is a protein important in blood clotting, and too much of it may make your blood thick and sticky, an effect that you could do without.

People with levels too high are twice as likely to die of a heart attack.

Taken together with other risk factors it could add to the urgency of specific therapy such as the use of omega-3 fatty acids that have been shown to reduce fibrinogen levels, and the use of aspirin for its anti-clotting activity.

Cardiovascular disease risk factor questions

Is your blood pressure over 120/80?   __Yes __No

Are you on any hypertension (high blood pressure) medication?   __Yes __No

Do you have a pre-existing cardiac condition?   __Yes __No

If so, are you under the care of a physician?   __Yes __No

Have you ever had a heart attack?   __Yes __No

Have you ever been told that you have angina?   __Yes __No

About cigarettes: Check those that apply.

___I never smoked ___I smoke a few cigarettes a day ___I smoke 1 pack per day

___I smoke 1 to 2 packs per day ___I smoke 2 or more packs per day

___I quit smoking ___I inhale ___I do not inhale ___I smoke cigars

___I smoke a pipe ___I am exposed to second hand smoke

___How many years have you smoked?____

___I have quit smoking in the last 5 years.

Have you ever had a total cholesterol test?   __Yes __No

    Date of last cholesterol test_____

    Is your total cholesterol greater than 200?   __Yes __No

    Is your LDL cholesterol level higher than 100 mg/dl?   __Yes __No

    Is your HDL cholesterol level lower than 40 mg/dl?   __Yes __No

Is your triglyceride level greater than 200?   __Yes __No

Do you have Diabetes?   __Yes __No

Would you describe the daily exercise you get as 'minimal or none'?   __Yes __No

Are you overweight?   __Yes __No

What is your weight in pounds?____

For a man: Does your waist at your belly button measure more than 40 inches?

__Yes __No

For a woman: Does your waist at your belly button measure more than 35 inches?

__Yes __No

What is your height in inches?_____

Are you subject to unusual stress?   __Yes __No

Do you drink more than two drinks a day?   __Yes __No

Did your grandfather, father, or brother have heart trouble or a heart attack before age 55?   __Yes __No

Did your grandmother, mother, or sister have heart trouble or a heart attack before age 65?   __Yes __No

Have you ever had any of the following blood tests: homocysteine, CRP, or fibrinogen?   __Yes __No

You have taken your first risk factor analysis. You will take more as you read this book, and, I repeat, when you finish you should bring this information to your physician for his or her analysis.

You must be proactive as regards your health. This is crucial. Your physician may not be able to take the time to assess you completely in this way. Help him or her by identifying all your risk factors. Then together you both can decide what positive risk factors demand corrective action or specific therapy. Again, I repeat, early disease detection and prevention is the name of the game, and it can't be done without a risk factor analysis—and a thorough and complete medical examination (the subject of my previous book: *The Patient's Guide to the Complete Medical Examination and the Prevention of Medical Errors*—(see appendix 1.)

CHAPTER 3

CANCER

Research shows that certain risk factors will increase your chance of getting cancer. Why one patient with these risk factors gets cancer and another patient with identical risk factors does not get cancer is unknown.

The good news is that most people who have the risk factors do not develop cancer, but you can not know if you are one of the lucky ones, so learn if you have them, and, if you do, take them seriously.

The most common risk factors for cancer are:

- Positive family history

- Chemicals

- Viruses and bacteria

- Ionizing radiation

- Hormones

- Obesity

- Poor diet

- Lack of exercise

- Sunlight

- Alcohol

- Tobacco

So, we will discuss the risk factors for the most common cancers.

Lung Cancer

In 1900, lung cancer was so rare it was a reportable disease. Then men started smoking heavily. By nineteen twenty, lung cancer in men began to mushroom.

Women started smoking heavily about 1920, and, sure enough, twenty years later, they joined the men.

Lung cancer kills more people than breast, colon, lymph, and prostate cancer combined. It is often diagnosed too late for cure, but a newer method, the spiral CT scan, may be changing this picture.

So, if you are a smoker check with your physician.

It has been estimated that eighty-seven percent of all lung cancer is due to cigarettes.

There are other risk factors, and they will be discussed, but cigarettes are an example of a single risk factor that is responsible for the vast majority of cases.

Lung cancer risk factors

Smoking

The risk increases the more you smoke, the earlier you started, and the deeper you inhale. If there is any good news here, it is that if you quit you reduce your risk. Even if you don't smoke, second hand smoke puts you at risk.

Asbestos and other chemicals

If you have been exposed to asbestos, coal products, vinyl chloride, or nickel chromate, you are at risk, and that risk is greater if you also smoke.

Radon gas

Uranium, found in the soil, rocks and water, slowly breaks down by radioactive decay and becomes part of the air we breathe (radon gas).

We should all test the radon levels in our home, because chronic exposure to radon gas is an important risk factor for lung cancer.

You can learn where to get the test by contacting your local health department, or the Environmental Protection Agency. You are at risk if radon exceeds recommended levels.

Lung infection

It is thought that a history of pneumonia or tuberculosis may, by virtue of its chronic scarring, put you at risk.

Heredity

It has been shown that there is a hereditary connection in lung cancer, so if you have a grandparent, father, mother, sister or brother who has had the disease, you are at risk even if you do not smoke.

Air pollution

If you have lived in a city known for its air pollution, you may be at greater risk in direct proportion to the length of time lived there.

Lung cancer risk factor questions

Do you smoke? __Yes __No

Have you quit smoking? __Yes __No

Are you exposed to second hand smoke? __Yes __No

Have you ever worked with asbestos? __Yes __No

Has your home ever been tested for radon? __Yes __No

If yes, did the radon test exceed recommended levels?   __Yes __No

Have you worked with chemicals?   __Yes __No

Have you ever worked in a mine?   __Yes __No

Do you smoke marijuana?   __Yes __No

Have you ever had pneumonia?   __Yes __No

Have you ever had tuberculosis?   __Yes __No

Have any of your grandparents, parents, brother, or sister had lung cancer?
                                                                   __Yes __No

Have you lived in a city known for its air pollution?   __Yes __No

Breast Cancer

Second only to lung cancer as a cause of cancer deaths in women, the prognosis is improving because of early detection.

Removal of the breast and all the lymph nodes (radical mastectomy) is rarely done today, this procedure being replaced by breast-sparing techniques.

About two-thousand men per year will get breast cancer.

The best screening test is a mammogram. Women in their forties should have a mammogram at least every two years. Those younger than forty who have significant risk factors should discuss with their physician whether to have mammograms earlier than forty and how often to have them.

Mammograms can identify a lump before it can be felt, and it can also demonstrate clusters of microcalcifications, which could mean cancer or a precancerous condition.

A biopsy is the only positive way to identify breast cancer.

Breast cancer risk factors

Previous breast cancer

If you have had a personal history of breast cancer, you face a higher risk of breast cancer in the other breast.

Age

Between the age of thirty to forty you have a low risk of breast cancer. The actual statistics are one in 233.

Eighty percent of breast cancers occur in woman over age fifty, and this gradually increases to one in eight by age eighty-five.

Family history

If you have had a mother, sister, or daughter who have had breast cancer before menopause you have an increased risk of developing the disease. The same is true for you if a male relative has had breast cancer. If a relative developed breast cancer before age fifty, your risk is doubled. And if two or more relatives have had breast cancer, your risk is even greater.

Five to ten percent of women have a hereditary form of the disease resulting from a mutation (change) in two genes (BRCA1 and BRCA2). These genes ordinarily are protective for cancer by making proteins that prevent cells from growing abnormally, but if one has the mutation, the reverse is true.

Those with the mutation are much more susceptible to breast cancer plus ovarian and colon cancer.

The possibility of a woman carrying this mutated gene is greater if there have been multiple cases of breast cancer in the family especially in more than one generation, or one or more family members have had breast and/or ovarian cancer, or a family member has had two different cancers at different sites.

If you have an Ashkenazi (Eastern European) Jewish background, you are also at increased risk for breast cancer.

Men who have a mutated BRCA1 gene have a greater risk of breast cancer and possibly prostate cancer.

Mutation in the BRCA2 gene has been associated with an increased risk for other cancers including lymphoma, melanoma, and upper gastrointestinal cancers involving the stomach, pancreas, gallbladder and bile ducts.

Obesity

Your breast cancer risk is increased if you have gained weight during your teen years, or after menopause.

If you have more body fat on the upper part of your body you are also at increased risk.

Menstrual cycle

You may have a greater breast cancer risk if your periods started before age twelve, and/or if you have had a late menopause. This may be related to longer exposure of breast tissue to estrogen.

Timing of pregnancy

If you have never been pregnant, or your first pregnancy occurred after age thirty you are at increased risk.

Radiation exposure

Radiation therapy to your chest area in early childhood will increase your risk for breast cancer. If the therapy was delivered when your breasts were developing your risk is higher.

Mammogram breast density

Dense breast tissue on a mammography study can make it difficult to read, thus possibly preventing accurate cancer interpretation. The density, by itself, has also been recognized as a cancer risk factor, but the reason for this slightly increased risk is not known.

If your breast tissue is too dense for accurate interpretation your physician may recommend other screening tests.

Hormone therapy

Four or more years of therapy with estrogen and progesterone therapy raises your risk for breast cancer, and can also make breast cancer interpretation on mammography more difficult.

The use of estrogen alone in postmenopausal woman does not increase breast cancer risk.

Birth control pills

There is an increased risk of breast cancer in premenopausal women who took birth control pills, and in women who took birth control pills for at least four years before their first pregnancy.

Smoking

This is a controversial issue. Some studies show no correlation, others do. This is just another reason to stop smoking.

Alcohol use

Your risk is increased by twenty percent if you drink more than one drink per day.

Breast cancer risk factor questions

Have you ever had breast cancer?   __Yes __No

Has your grandmother, mother, or sister ever had breast cancer?   __Yes __No

Have two or more members of your family in different generations had breast and or ovarian cancer?   __Yes __No

Have you gained weight in your teen years or after menopause?   __Yes __No

Have you ever been pregnant?   __Yes __No

Did you have your first child after age 30?   __Yes __No

Have you ever been exposed to radiation therapy to your chest during early child-hood or adolescence?   __Yes __No

Have you ever been told that your mammogram showed dense breast tissue?
                                                                      __Yes __No

Have you taken estrogen and progesterone for more than four years?   __Yes __No

Have you taken birth control pills during your menstruating years, or have you taken birth control pills for four years before your first pregnancy?   __Yes __No

Do you smoke?   __Yes __No

Do you drink alcohol more than one drink per day?   __Yes __No

Skin Cancer

There are three forms of skin cancer:

Basal cell carcinoma—grows slowly and does not spread to distant sites. This form of skin cancer is highly treatable, especially when caught early.

Squamous cell carcinoma—grows slowly, but can spread to distant sites (metastasis). This form is highly treatable unless caught late.

Melanoma—the most serious form of the disease involves deeper skin layers, and has the greatest potential to metastasize.

All these cancers are on the rise, so if you have risk factors for skin cancer you and your physician should decide the frequency of a full skin review.

Exposure to sun (ultraviolet radiation) is the most common cause of skin cancer.

The good news is that all forms of skin cancer can be cured if caught early.

Skin cancer risk factors

Previous history of skin cancer

If you previously have had skin cancer, you are at greater risk for a second episode.

Precancerous skin lesions

Sun-damaged sites are often the area where actinic keratoses (a pre-malignant lesion) can form. These are rough, scaly pink to brown patches.

Blonde or red haired people are most susceptible; blacks are rarely affected.

Sun exposure

If you are a sun worshipper, you are at increased risk for skin cancer especially if you do not use sunscreen.

Suntans, either by exposure to sun or tanning baths, put you at increased risk also.

Sunburn

Sunburn damages your skin, putting you at increased risk for skin cancer.

Light-skinned features

Less skin pigment provides less protection against ultra-violet radiation, which puts you at greater risk.

Freckles, blond or red hair and light-colored eyes also put you at greater risk for skin cancer.

Family history

A positive family history of skin cancer in a grandparent, parent, or sibling may put you at greater risk.

Numerous moles

If you have many moles you are at increased risk, and you should have them evaluated at least once per year.

Chemical exposure

Such exposure increases your risk for skin cancer.

Skin cancer risk factor questions

Have you ever been diagnosed with skin cancer?	__Yes __No
Have you ever been told you have actinic keratoses?	__Yes __No
Have you been told you have fair (light) skin?	__Yes __No
Do you have red or blond hair?	__Yes __No
Do you have freckles?	__Yes __No
Do you sunburn easily?	__Yes __No
Have you had severe, blistering sunburns, especially as a child?	__Yes __No
Do you get excessive sun exposure?	__Yes __No
Have you lived in a sunny high-altitude climate?	__Yes __No
Has one of your grandparents, parents or a brother or sister ever had skin cancer?	__Yes __No
Do you have many moles?	__Yes __No
Have you been exposed to environmental chemicals or herbicides?	__Yes __No

Ovarian Cancer

This disease is difficult to diagnose in its early stages, because the cancer has room to grow before it impacts adjacent organs, and symptoms can be vague and non diagnostic.

Your chance of survival is greater the earlier the cancer is found.

It has recently been found that certain symptoms may be indicative of early ovarian cancer. These include pelvic discomfort, pelvic pain, frequent urge to urinate, abdominal swelling or bloating, diarrhea, constipation, indigestion, nausea, gas, loss of appetite, weight loss or gain. You should see your physician early if you have any of these symptoms.

Ovarian cancer risk factors

Family history

If your mother, daughter or sister has had ovarian cancer you have five percent risk of getting the disease.

BRCA1 or BRCA2 gene

These genes are responsible for about five to ten percent of ovarian cancers.

Pregnancy

At least one pregnancy puts you at lower risk.

Birth control pills

The use of birth control pills put you at lower risk.

Infertility

Infertility puts you at greater risk. This applies if you have had difficulty conceiving or if you have never conceived.

Ovarian cyst

An ovarian cyst that develops after the menopause has a greater chance of becoming malignant.

Hormone replacement therapy

Woman who have not had a hysterectomy, and have been on postmenopausal hormone replacement therapy for five or more years, have a significantly higher rate of ovarian cancer.

Obesity

Women who have been obese in their late teen years have an increased risk for ovarian cancer before the menopause.

Ovarian Cancer risk factor questions

Do you have/had a grandmother, mother, sister, or daughter with Ovarian Cancer?

__Yes __No

Do you or your family members carry the BRCA1 or 2 gene?   __Yes __No

Are you post-menopausal?   __Yes __No

Have you ever been pregnant?   __Yes __No

Have you taken birth control pills?   __Yes __No

Do you have a history of infertility?   __Yes __No

Have you been diagnosed with an ovarian cyst?   __Yes __No

Do you take/have taken hormone replacement therapy after menopause?

__Yes __No

Were you overweight in your teenage years?   __Yes __No

Prostate Cancer

The incidence of prostate cancer increases as men age. By the time men reach age eighty, it is estimated that almost eighty percent will have prostate cancer. Luckily, it is of the form that stays local in most instances, but that is not always the case.

African Americans have a higher incidence of cancer than Caucasians.

The average risk patient should have screening by a rectal examination and a prostate specific antigen (PSA) blood test starting at age fifty.

High risk patients with a strong family history, or African Americans should start screening studies at age forty.

Prostate cancer risk factors

Age

Although prostate cancer can develop in the forties, most commonly it develops over age fifty. As one ages the possibility of prostate cancer increases.

Race

African-American men have a higher risk of developing prostate cancer at an earlier age. They also have a higher risk of dying from it. The reasons are not clear.

Family history

If your father or brother has had prostate cancer, you are at greater risk.

Diet

Those men who eat a high fat diet (milk and meat) are at greater risk, possibly because fat increases the production of testosterone that can stimulate prostate cancer cell growth.

Obesity

Men who are overweight have been shown to be more likely to develop a more aggressive form of prostate cancer.

Prostate cancer risk factor questions

Are you Caucasian (white)?   __Yes __No

And are you over fifty years of age?   __Yes __No

Are you black?   __Yes __No

And are you over forty years of age?   __Yes __No

Has your father or brother had cancer of the prostate?   __Yes __No

Have any other relatives had prostate cancer?   __Yes __No

Would you say you eat a diet high in fat (butter, meat, sausage, bacon, cakes, pastries, take-away foods)?   __Yes __No

Do you drink more than two glasses of milk per day?   __Yes __No

Do you get regular exercise?   __Yes __No

Are you overweight?   __Yes __No

Colon Cancer

Colon cancer, including rectal cancer, is the second-leading cause of cancer deaths. Only lung cancer is responsible for more cancer deaths.

The good news is that the great majority of colon cancers start out as tiny polyps that can be easily removed by colonoscopy. In their early stages, polyps cause no symptoms. That is why screening is so important. If polyps are allowed to continue to grow they may eventually cause symptoms such as rectal bleeding, change in bowel habits, abdominal pain or gas and cramps. But by then, it may be too late for a cure.

You should discuss the time for screening with your personal physician.

Colon cancer risk factors

Age

Ninety percent of colon cancer occurs after age fifty.

Inflammatory intestinal conditions

Colon cancer risk increases if you have Crohn's disease or ulcerative colitis, both inflammatory diseases of the colon.

Family history

Your risk for colon cancer is greater if you have a grandparent, parent, or brother or sister who has the disease.

Familial hereditary polyposis is a rare condition where multiple polyps grow in the colon lining. If left untreated you will most certainly develop colon cancer by age forty.

An Ashkenazi Jew has a greater likelihood of developing colon cancer.

Diet

If you eat a high fat, low fiber diet you are at greater risk for colon cancer

Inactivity

Inactivity puts you at greater risk for colon cancer possibly because when you are inactive, waste remains in the colon longer. Regular physical exercise promotes bowel regularity, which reduces the risk.

Smoking

It has been estimated that smoking is responsible for one in ten colon cancers.

Alcohol

More than two drinks per day may increase your risk for colon cancer.

Diabetes

Diabetics have a forty percent greater risk for colon cancer.

Colon cancer risk factors questions

Are you more than 50 years of age?   __Yes __No

Have you ever been diagnosed with Ulcerative colitis or Crohn's disease?   __Yes __No

Have you ever had colon/rectal polyps or cancer?   __Yes __No

Has a grandparent, parent, brother or sister, or child ever had colon cancer?   __Yes __No

Are you an Ashkenazi Jew (from Eastern Europe)?   __Yes __No

Familial adenomatous polyposis is a hereditary disorder where multiple polyps line your colon. Has anyone in your family suffered from this condition?   __Yes __No

Is your diet low in fiber and high in fat?   __Yes __No

Are you inactive—rarely exercise?   __Yes __No

Do you smoke?   __Yes __No

Do you consume more than one alcoholic drink per day?   __Yes __No

Are you diabetic?   __Yes __No

Have you had a colonoscopy?   __Yes __No

If so when? _____

Pancreatic Cancer

The pancreas secretes hormones that control carbohydrate metabolism and enzymes that aid digestion. It is an organ that lies horizontally behind the stomach.

If it becomes cancerous it has room to grow, so symptoms often do not develop until it has already spread.

Most pancreatic cancers occur after age sixty-five.

African-Americans have a higher risk of pancreatic cancer.

More men than women are at risk.

Pancreatic cancer risk factors

Cigarette smoking

Cigarette smoke is associated with one-third of pancreatic cancers. A smoker is three times as likely to develop pancreatic cancer as a non smoker.

Diabetes

Diabetes increases your risk for pancreatic cancer. How it is related to the pancreas' problems with carbohydrate metabolism in diabetes is not known.

Diet

Those who do not eat fruits and vegetables and eat a diet high in fat have an increased risk.

Obesity

Again, this risk factor makes itself felt.

Hereditary pancreatitis

Thankfully, this is a very rare genetic condition where painful attacks of pancreatitis (inflammation of the pancreas) occur. These patients are at higher risk for cancer most certainly because of the recurrent pancreatic attacks.

Exposure to petroleum products

Those who work with gasoline and other chemical petroleum products are at higher risk.

Pancreatic risk factor questions

Do you smoke?   __Yes __No

Do you have diabetes?   __Yes __No

Do you eat a high fat diet and rarely eat fruits and vegetables?   __Yes __No

Have you had repeated bouts of pancreatitis?   __Yes __No

Do you work with gasoline or other chemical petroleum products?   __Yes __No

CHAPTER 4

STROKE
(CEREBROVASCULAR
DISEASE)

Stroke ranks third as a cause of death and disability; it occurs when the blood supply to a portion of your brain is interrupted either by a clot in a brain blood vessel or hemorrhage from a brain blood vessel. The disruption to the flow of blood to the brain tissue results in brain cell death within minutes.

If treatment for a stroke can be started rapidly, there is a better chance of a full recovery.

The incidence of stroke is declining, probably because there has been better control of the risk factors for stroke—smoking and high blood pressure.

There are no differences in the risk factors for stroke as there are for heart disease (heart attack). This is true, of course, because we are dealing with blood vessels, and the risk factors we do not follow that impact our blood vessels impact them all regardless of where they are in the body, including the brain.

So, your risk is greater if there is a member of our family who has had a stroke; if you get older; if you are African American (probably because of the higher incidence of high blood pressure); if you have an elevated blood pressure; if your LDL cholesterol is too high; if your HDL cholesterol is too low; if you smoke; if you have diabetes; if you are obese; if you do not exercise; if you have an elevated homocysteine level, c-reactive protein, or fibrinogen.

Other stroke risk factors

Cardiac disease

Stroke risk increases if you have had a previous heart attack, heart failure, abnormal functioning of the valves of your heart, infection on a heart valve (endocarditis), and atrial fibrillation (an irregularity of the heart rhythm).

The reason these problems can cause a stroke is because of the tendency for clots to form in a heart thusly diseased. These clots can then break off and travel to the brain.

Previous stroke

A risk for a repeat stroke is greater if one has had a previous stroke, or has had a mini-stroke also known as a transient cerebral ischemic attack (ischemia meaning lack of blood or oxygen).

Smoker: Age greater than thirty-five and taking birth control pills

If you are a smoker and are over age thirty-five and you take birth control pills, you are at increased risk for stroke, although the newer low-dose pills carry considerable less risk.

Sleep Apnea

If you have moderate to severe sleep apnea (restless sleep and more than twenty breathing pauses per hour usually due to blockage of the windpipe), you have a greater risk for stroke.

Stroke risk factor questions

Same as cardiac risk factor questions plus:

Have you been diagnosed with a heart attack, heart failure, heart valve problems, endocarditis, atrial fibrillation?   __Yes __No

Have you ever had a stroke or transient cerebral ischemic attack?   __Yes __No

Are you thirty-five or older, smoke and take birth control pills?   __Yes __No

Do you have moderate to severe obstructive sleep apnea?   __Yes __No

CHAPTER 5

CHRONIC LOWER RESPIRATORY DISEASE (EMPHYSEMA, CHRONIC BRONCHITIS)

Progressive damage to the air sacs of the lung and small bronchial tubes results in an obstruction to the flow of air when you exhale. The damage occurs slowly, so the disease may be fairly well advanced by the time you become symptomatic.

Long time cigarette use is the most common cause. Likewise cigarette use, or recurrent bouts of acute bronchitis (infection of the bronchial tube lining), can result in a chronic bronchitis.

Chronic bronchitis is diagnosed when you have a productive cough lasting three months in two successive years.

Chronic lower respiratory disease risk factors

Tobacco smoke

Far and away, the greatest risk factor for this illness is smoking. Cigarettes are incriminated the most, but the risk is present also with cigars, pipe and second hand smoke. The more years you smoke and the amount you smoke is directly proportional to increasing risk.

Age

Emphysema is rarely seen before age forty except for one rare exception (see heredity below).

Exposure to air pollution, chemical fumes and dust

These environmental and occupational factors slowly irritate and damage the lungs.

Asthma

Some individuals with asthma can develop emphysema.

Heredity

Alpha-1 antitrypsin (AAT) deficiency can cause emphysema. AAT is a protein that is made by the liver. One of its functions is to protect the lungs. Because of a gene problem, some of us have very little or none of it, and if that is the case we will get emphysema usually before age forty. Needless to say, people who have this genetic defect and who still smoke are asking for trouble.

Low birth weight and prematurity

Premature infants often have lung disease (premature interstitial emphysema). If they survive, they may develop a chronic lung problem.

Chronic lower respiratory disease risk factor questions

Do you smoke cigarettes?   __Yes __No

How long have you smoked?_____

Have you been exposed to chemicals, industrial smoke, dusts from mining?

                                                                __Yes __No

Has anyone in your family who did not smoke ever have chronic obstructive lung disease (emphysema)?   __Yes __No

Have you ever had allergies or asthma?   __Yes __No

Do you have a history of a low birth weight or prematurity?   __Yes __No

CHAPTER 6

UNINTENTIONAL INJURIES (ACCIDENTS)

Injuries in all categories will be discussed below.

Accident risk factors

Traffic accidents

The number one killer by far—43,200 per year.

Falls

There are 14,900 deaths per year, including falls of all kinds and in all places—indoor and out.

The older you are, the less of a fall is required to kill you.

Poisoning by solids and liquids

There are 8,600 deaths per year. This category includes, mushrooms, shellfish, chemical poisons, medication and illegal drug overdoses.

Drowning

Four thousand per year die a watery death either through swimming, water sports, boating and yes, bathing.

Fire

Three thousand seven hundred per year die of fire or smoke, and most of the fires are caused by cigarettes. Now add to this statistic the fact that cigarettes are a prominent risk factor for heart disease, stroke, cancer, and lung disease, the leading causes of medical deaths, and it raises the question of why human beings would expose themselves to such risk.

Addiction is indeed a powerful force.

Suffocation

Three thousand three hundred people per year die of food or other objects obstructing respiration. Eating and drinking alcohol together, or biting off large pieces increases your risk for suffocation

Guns

Fifteen hundred people per year—mostly young males aged fourteen to twenty-five—are killed by guns.

As long as we have the second amendment, I guess that statistic will persist and the victims will keep getting younger.

Interestingly, in many countries of the world this statistic will not find itself in the top twenty leading causes of death because of restrictive gun laws.

Poisoning by gas

Seven hundred people per year die of carbon monoxide resulting from an automobile or a faulty heating or cooking appliance.

Medical and surgical complications and misadventures

It has been estimated that there are five hundred deaths per year in the category of medical and surgical complications and misadventures.

Machinery

Farm machinery accidents result in 350 deaths per year.

Accident risk factor questions

Do you use your seat belt every time you drive?	__Yes __No
Have you driven after drinking alcohol?	__Yes __No
Have you consistently exceeded speed limits?	__Yes __No
Have you driven while on the influence of drugs?	__Yes __No
Do you have trouble walking?	__Yes __No
Do you use a cane?	__Yes __No
Do you use a ladder?	__Yes __No
Do you have nonskid mats in showers and tubs?	__Yes __No
Do you read labels carefully?	__Yes __No
Do you work with chemicals?	__Yes __No
Do you swim alone?	__Yes __No
Do you wear a life preserver when you are in a boat?	__Yes __No
Do you have a working fire-extinguisher in your home?	__Yes __No
Do you have smoke detectors near bedrooms?	__Yes __No
Do you smoke in bed?	__Yes __No
Do you drink alcohol and eat at the same time?	__Yes __No
Do you swallow large bites of food?	__Yes __No
Do you have a gun in your home?	__Yes __No
Do you have carbon monoxide detectors near bedrooms?	__Yes __No

Do you work in agriculture, mining, or construction?   __Yes __No

CHAPTER 7

DIABETES MELLITUS

To review: Type 1 diabetes effects younger patients and is an autoimmune disease. Your immune system turns against your insulin-producing cells of the pancreas resulting in the inability to make insulin, which has to be replaced by injectable insulin for you to stay alive.

Type 2 diabetes is a condition resulting from the inability of your body to process sugar correctly. This condition is increasing because it results from the obesity epidemic.

The control of diabetes depends upon a compliant, educated patient.

Diabetes risk factors

Age

The risk for diabetes increases with age, especially after forty-five years. This is probably due to weight gain and decreasing physical activity as one gets older. This type of adult onset diabetes is seen in younger children and young adults, most certainly for the same two reasons.

Weight

If you are a male and your waist measurement exceeds forty inches, and if you are female and your waist measurement exceeds thirty-five inches, you have increased your risk for diabetes.

Even a slight weight gain puts you at higher risk.

Family history

Your risk for diabetes increases with each family member who has developed the disease.

Cardiac risk factors

If you should have cardiac risk factors such as a low HDL, a high LDL and hypertension, then it is urgent that everything be done to improve those results and pay strict attention to all diabetes risk factors.

Prediabetes

A 'borderline' blood sugar elevation often means that you have reached a prediabetic state. This can be reversed, and everything should be done to reverse it so that it doesn't evolve into full-blown diabetes.

Inactivity

Exercise can reduce your blood sugar, control your weight, lower your blood pressure, reduce your total cholesterol and LDL cholesterol, raise your HDL cholesterol—all beneficial effects in preventing diabetes which has a negative effect on the vascular system.

A thirty minute daily walk can reduce the onset of diabetes by fifty percent.

Poor diet

Junk food, sugary food, high fat foods promote the development of diabetes. They also cause you to gain weight—another diabetic risk factor.

Race

Diabetes is more common in African Americans, Native Americans, Asian Americans, Hispanic Americans and Pacific Islanders.

Gestational diabetes

If you were pregnant and never had diabetes before, but have had a high blood sugar during pregnancy, you have gestational diabetes. Why this happens we're not sure, but it is possible that hormones from the placenta, which help the baby develop, also may block the effect of the mother's insulin.

This is known as insulin resistance. This may affect the baby in terms of future obesity and development of diabetes.

The good news is that in virtually all instances, after the pregnancy, the gestational diabetic state resolves, but a mother to whom this happens should remain alert and pay attention to risk factors for diabetes as they may be more prone to its future development.

Diabetes risk factor questions

Are you 45 years of age or older?   __Yes __No

Does your waist (around your belly button measure more than 40 inches if you are a man and thirty-five inches if you are a woman?); would you say you have a pot belly?   __Yes __No

Is there any diabetes in your family?   __Yes __No

Is your HDL cholesterol under 35?   __Yes __No

Is your triglyceride level more than 200?   __Yes __No

Have you been told that you have high blood pressure?   __Yes __No

Have you ever been told that your blood glucose level is higher than normal, but not high enough to be diagnosed with diabetes?   __Yes __No

Are you inactive—do you exercise infrequently?   __Yes __No

Would you say you have a poor diet; you miss meals, eat on the run, too much junk food, too much sugar?   __Yes __No

Are you African American, Hispanic American, Native American, Asian American, or Pacific Islander?   __Yes __No

When you were pregnant was your blood sugar elevated, or were you diagnosed with gestational diabetes?   __Yes __No

CHAPTER 8

INFLUENZA (FLU) AND PNEUMONIA

Ten to twenty percent of the population may get flu during the flu season extending from November through March.

The best prophylaxis is an annual flu vaccine. One contraindication to flu vaccine use is if you are allergic to eggs, since egg products are used in the manufacture of the flu vaccine.

If you are pregnant during the flu season you should take the flu vaccine if your physician approves, although pregnant women should avoid the nasal flu mist (LAIV) as it has not been approved for use during pregnancy.

There is a pneumonia vaccine as well. Your doctor will advise you if you should take this vaccine.

There are other things that can be done to help avoid the flu:

- Clean your hands often.

- Avoid close contact with those that have the flu.

- Keep your hands away from your eyes, nose, or mouth.

- Stay home if you are sick.

- If you sneeze or cough, cover your nose and mouth with a tissue.

Influenza (Flu) and Pneumonia risk factors

Age

Highest risk patients are infants, children and senior citizens. Of course, anyone is susceptible. Those at highest risk are more susceptible to complications of flu such as pneumonia.

Chronic illness

Those with chronic illnesses such as heart disease, lung disease, kidney disease, or diabetes have the greatest risk for flu complications.

Medications

If you take medications that suppress your immune system, you are at higher risk for flu and its complications.

Workplace

If you work in a crowded environment and come in contact with many people, you are at greater risk for getting the flu.

Influenza and pneumonia risk factor questions

Are you fifty years of age or older?   __Yes __No

Do you have asthma or heart or lung or kidney problems?   __Yes __No

Do you have any other chronic disease requiring close medical supervision?
                                                                                  __Yes __No

Do you take any medications that suppress your immune system?   __Yes __No

Do you get a yearly flu shot (flu vaccine)?   __Yes __No

Have you ever had a pneumonia shot (pnemococcal vaccine)?   __Yes __No

CHAPTER 9

ALZHEIMER'S DISEASE

Alois Alzheimer was a German physician and neuropsychiatrist who described an unusual case *"eine eigenartige Erkrankung der Hirnrinde"* (a peculiar disease of the cerebral cortex).

The patient was a woman in her fifties who had all the clinical and pathological features of a disease that would soon be known as Alzheimer's disease.

In those days, people did not live as long as they do today. There was senility of old age, and there was a rare younger case, like Alzheimer's patient who became progressively more disoriented, suffered increasing impairment of memory, and lost the ability to read and to write.

When she died, a pathological study was made of the patient's brain and the characteristic feature of what is now known as Alzheimer's disease was described.

We now live longer, and Alzheimer's disease strikes fifty percent more of us if we live long enough. Can we do anything to prevent it?

Alzheimer's disease risk factors

Age

As you get older you are at increasing risk. Between the ages of 65 and 74, five percent of people have Alzheimer's disease. By age 85, fifty percent are afflicted.

Heredity

Alzheimer's disease developing between the age of forty and sixty is genetic in origin. It is not clear if there is a genetic origin in late onset Alzheimer's.

Cardiac risk factors

If you have cardiac risk factors such as an elevated cholesterol and high blood pressure, it has been suggested that you are more prone to Alzheimer's disease.

Head injury

Some studies have incriminated a prior severe head injury with future Alzheimer's disease. Former boxers have developed a condition known as dementia pugilistica, which is pathologically similar to Alzheimer's disease.

Physical, mental and social factors

Evidence is accumulating that if you are physically active, mentally active and socially outgoing, you are at lesser risk for Alzheimer's disease.

Alzheimer's disease risk factor questions

Are you 80 years old or older?   __Yes __No

Are you 65 to 80 years old?   __Yes __No

Has one of your parents or brother or sister had Alzheimer's disease?   __Yes __No

Have you had heart disease, high blood pressure, high cholesterol?   __Yes __No

Have you had a head injury with unconsciousness?   __Yes __No

What is your highest educational level?

___High school ___Trade school___College ___Graduate school

Would you say you engage in continuous learning?   __Yes __No

Do you exercise regularly?   __Yes __No

CHAPTER 10

KIDNEY DISEASE (NEPHRITIS OR NEPHROSIS)

The main function of your kidneys is to filter waste products out of your blood and eliminate them through the urine. The loss of this filtering function develops very slowly, and you will not know that it is happening until you have lost about seventy-five percent of your kidney function. At this stage, the main goal is to prevent further decline so as not to necessitate kidney dialysis or kidney transplant.

Kidney disease risk factors

High blood pressure

Untreated high blood pressure can cause slow, progressive kidney damage.

Prostate enlargement

Prostate enlargement affects every man over aged fifty to some degree. If the enlargement becomes severe, it is possible that there can be enough back pressure on the kidneys to damage them significantly.

This is one of the reasons men with prostate enlargement should be followed closely by a physician.

Diabetes Mellitus

Uncontrolled diabetes can lead to progressive kidney failure.

Immune disorders

Scleroderma or lupus erythematosis, both autoimmune disorders, can involve and adversely affect the kidneys.

Nephritis or Nephrosis

There are numerous medical causes of nephritis or nephrosis, and they can lead to kidney failure.

Congenital kidney disease

There are some congenital kidney diseases that can result in adult kidney failure. An example is polycystic kidneys, where enlarging cysts gradually replace functioning kidney tissue.

Bladder outlet obstruction

Besides prostate enlargement, there are other causes of bladder outlet obstruction such as prostate cancer, scarring of the urethra, bladder stones, surgical injury, or medications such as nasal decongestants and antihistamines.

Non-steroidal anti-inflammatory medicine.

The chronic use of these medications, and on rare occasions, just one pill can cause kidney failure.

Kidney disease risk factor questions

Do you have high blood pressure or heart disease?   __Yes __No

Have you ever been told that you have an enlarged prostate?   __Yes __No

Do you have diabetes?   __Yes __No

Have you ever been diagnosed with an immune disorder such as lupus erythematosis or scleroderma?   __Yes __No

Have you ever been diagnosed with heart trouble or hardening of the arteries?
__Yes __No

Have you ever been told that you had nephritis or nephrosis?   __Yes __No

Were you born with kidney problem?   __Yes __No

Have you ever been told that you have a bladder outlet obstruction?   __Yes __No

Do you take aspirin, non-steroidal anti-inflammatory medicine every day? (Motrin, Advil, Tylenol)?   __Yes __No

CHAPTER 11

SEPTICEMIA
(SEVERE INFECTION)

Septicemia refers to bacterial invasion of the blood stream, the so-called "blood poisoning." Clearly this is a dangerous condition because the bacteria can thrive in this favorable environment and liberate toxins which can cause low blood pressure, organ failure and death.

Thankfully this is not often seen in young, healthy individuals, but is not uncommon in the elderly.

Septicemia risk factors

Predisposing factors include any chronic illness such as diabetes, cirrhosis of the liver, cancer and cancer treatment with chemotherapy.

The use of invasive devices as part of therapy—intravenous lines, endotracheal tubes, urinary catheters, blood vessel catheters and drainage tubes have also been incriminated. These devices can pave the way for bacterial invasion of the blood stream.

Septicemia risk factor questions

Do you have a chronic medical illness requiring intense therapy and medical care?   __Yes __No

Have you recently had an invasive device used in therapy (drainage tubes, intravenous lines, catheters)?   __Yes __No

CHAPTER 12

SUICIDE

Thirty two thousand people per year die by their own hand, an average of one every eighteen minutes.

Males are four times as likely to commit suicide then females.

There are 730,000 attempts made per year, and women attempt suicide three times as often as men.

Suicides in teens are increasing to the extent that suicide is the third leading cause of deaths amongst teens, after accidents and homicide.

Clearly suicide is the ultimate manifestation of depression, but there are other factors as well: loss, impulsivity, broken homes, abuse, aggression, traumatic experience, self destructive behavior, serious chronic illness.

Suicide risk factors

Male over aged sixty-five

Men commit suicide more than women and it is more common after age sixty-five.

Previous attempt

A previous suicide attempt suggests it might be tried again.

Planning suicide

Making plans for suicide or thinking about methods or verbalizing the desire should be taken seriously.

Family history

Suicide attempts or successful suicides are more common where there has been a family history of suicide or a family history of major depression.

Anniversaries

Suicide attempts are more common on special anniversaries that have great personal significance.

Financial difficulties

A serious reduction of one's standard of living as a result of job loss or financial setback may prompt a suicide attempt.

Separation, divorce, sudden widowed status

A sudden change in one's social status may prompt a suicide attempt.

Sudden alcohol or drug use

A sudden immersion into alcohol or drug use can be caused by depression or anxiety due to a change in one's personal or social or financial status, and could presage disaster.

Suicide risk factor questions

Are you being treated for depression?   __Yes __No

Are you a male over aged sixty-five?   __Yes __No

Have you previously attempted suicide?   __Yes __No

Has anyone in your immediate family committed suicide?   __Yes __No

Is there an anniversary that has a particular and sad significance that you dwell on?   __Yes __No

Have you experienced a painful reduction in your financial status recently?
                                                                          __Yes __No

Have you experienced a sudden and recent separation, divorce, or death of a spouse?   __Yes __No

Have you recently turned to drugs or alcohol in an attempt to relieve anxiety or depression based upon a recent traumatic event?   __Yes __No

CHAPTER 13

LIVER DISEASE (CHRONIC HEPATITIS, CIRRHOSIS)

Hepatitis is an inflammation of the liver caused by viruses, drugs, or alcohol. There are three forms of viral hepatitis that are clinically significant:

1. Hepatitis A is spread by oral-fecal contact or the ingestion of contaminated raw shellfish. This form of hepatitis does not become chronic or lead to cirrhosis of the liver, a chronic state of advanced liver damage.

2. Hepatitis B is spread by contact with infected blood, (a risk for healthcare workers); through heterosexual and homosexual sex; by sharing needles through drug use; or the use of tattoo needles. All blood transfusions are tested for this virus eliminating this as a cause of transmission. From 0.5 percent to 10 percent of those infected can become chronic carriers.

3. Hepatitis C has a similar mode of transmission as hepatitis B. All blood transfusions are also tested for the virus. Eighty-five percent of patients who have hepatitis C carry the virus chronically and some can advance into clinically acute disease and even liver failure, but most instances of acute infection are clinically undetectable.

Hepatitis A, B, C risk factors

Foreign travel

One has to be careful eating food in rural areas of developing countries, but that does not mean you can not pick up the virus in a five-star hotel.

Hepatitis A is prevalent in Mexico, South America's Amazon Basin, Pacific Islands, Africa, Asia, and the Middle East.

Hepatitis A vaccine and immune globulin are recommended for all travelers to those countries.

Sexual activity

You are at increased risk for Hepatitis A, B if you are a sexually active and do not use condoms.

Illicit drug use

You are at increased risk for Hepatitis A, B, C, if you have used illegal injectable or oral drugs or nasal spray.

Work setting

You are at risk if you work in a laboratory or clinical setting where you could be exposed to human blood or any of the three viruses.

You can be exposed to Hepatitis A If you work in childcare and do not practice good hand hygiene.

Home setting

If you live in a household with a hepatitis carrier you are at risk unless vaccinated.

Blood transfusion

You are at risk if you received a blood transfusion prior to 1970 before they started testing for hepatitis B.

You are at risk if you received a blood transfusion prior to 1992 before they started testing for hepatitis C.

Organ transplant

You are at increased risk for hepatitis B if you received an organ transplant before 1992.

Clotting factors

You are at increased risk for hepatitis B if you received blood clotting factors before 1987.

Alcohol

Alcohol can cause a form of hepatitis. Four or more drinks per day for men, and two or more drinks per day for women will increase one's risk for liver damage.

Women are more susceptible to the effects of alcohol.

Hepatitis risk factor questions

Have you recently traveled to Mexico, South America, Pacific Islands, Asia, Africa, or the Middle East?   __Yes __No

Are you sexually active and do not use condoms?   __Yes __No

Have you used illegal intravenous, oral, or nasal spray drugs?   __Yes __No

Do you work in a laboratory or clinical setting where you are exposed to blood?
                                                                                 __Yes __No

Do you live in a household where there is a hepatitis carrier?   __Yes __No

Have you received a blood transfusion prior to 1970 before they started testing for Hepatitis B?   __Yes __No

Have you received a blood transfusion prior to 1992 when they started testing for Hepatitis C?   __Yes __No

Have you received an organ transplant before 1992?   __Yes __No

If you are a man do you drink four or more alcohol drinks per day, and if you are a woman do you drink two or more alcohol drinks per day?   __Yes __No

CHAPTER 14

ESSENTIAL HYPERTENSION (HIGH BLOOD PRESSURE)

Blacks have a higher incidence and get hypertension at a younger age than whites. Complications of an elevated blood pressure (heart attack, stroke, kidney failure) are more common in blacks.

The great majority of patients who have hypertension have a form known as essential hypertension. This form can be controlled by a compliant patient, lifestyle changes including weight loss, exercise, low salt diet, stress reduction, medication, and regular follow-up under the control of a physician. Hypertension that can not be controlled in spite of these measures, demands a careful search for unusual causes.

Hypertension risk factors

Race

More common in blacks than whites, but all races are susceptible.

Age

Blood pressure rises with age, and is more common in men. Women are more prone to elevated blood pressure after the menopause.

Overweight

The heavier you are the greater the amount of blood necessary to meet your bodies requirements, and as this blood volume increases so does your blood pressure.

Lack of exercise

This increases your risk for obesity. Also, with inactivity, you are de-conditioned and your heart rate beats faster necessitating more work with each beat increasing the force on your arteries.

Tobacco

Cigarettes, or other forms of tobacco, injure the lining of your arteries narrowing them and raising blood pressure.

Alcohol

Excessive drinking can damage your cardiovascular system.

Sodium (salt)

Too much salt in your diet can lead to fluid retention which increases blood volume and raises blood pressure. Some people are salt sensitive, exaggerating this effect.

Low potassium intake

Some studies have linked low potassium intake to a higher blood pressure. Potassium and sodium work together to balance the sodium in cells, so a lack of potassium can result in an increase in sodium in your cells resulting in a higher blood pressure.

Stress

Stress can cause a temporary rise in blood pressure and is thought to contribute to its development.

Some people have a form of blood pressure elevation known as white coat hypertension. Their blood pressure is much higher in doctor's offices than in their home. This in itself may have long term effects.

Other chronic medical conditions

If you have diabetes, kidney trouble, elevated cholesterol, or sleep apnea, you are at risk for an elevated blood pressure.

Essential hypertension risk factor questions

Are you African-American?   __Yes __No

Are you past your menopause (woman only)?   __Yes __No

Do you consider yourself to be overweight?   __Yes __No

Would you say you are inactive and rarely exercise?   __Yes __No

Do you smoke tobacco?   __Yes __No

Do you drink more than two alcohol drinks a day?   __Yes __No

Are you a heavy salt eater?   __Yes __No

Fish, fruits, fruit and vegetable juices, low fat yogurt, nuts, beans, potatoes, are rich in potassium. Do you eat these foods?   __Yes __No

Would you say that you have a significant amount of stress in your home or work life?   __Yes __No

Do you diabetes, kidney trouble, have high cholesterol, sleep apnea?   __Yes __No

CHAPTER 15

OSTEOPOROSIS

Osteoporosis means "porous bone." Bone is progressively lost over time, gradually becoming more brittle until one of your bones breaks.

The entire process is usually asymptomatic and the fracture may be the first manifestation of the disease.

Bones can become so brittle that even a sneeze, cough, bending over, or the simple act of lifting something may result in a fracture.

The hip and spine and wrist are mostly affected, but any bone may be involved.

It is estimated to affect 28,000,000 Americans and is responsible for 1,500,000 fractures per year.

Women are principally affected, but osteoporosis can strike men as well.

The reason for the brittleness is the gradual loss of calcium from bone. Much can be done to prevent this disorder.

Osteoporosis risk factors

Age and sex

Your risk for osteoporosis increases as you age.

At menopause, woman's estrogen level drops and this promotes more bone loss.

Also as men age, their testosterone level drops increasing their risk as well.

From age seventy-five on the rate of osteoporosis in women and men is equal.

Race

Whites and Southeast Asians have the highest incidence of osteoporosis. Hispanics and blacks have a lesser, but not insignificant risk.

Body size

A thin man or woman with a small body frame has a higher incidence. This probably reflects the fact that small bones, affected by osteoporosis, are likely to reach a fracture point sooner than large bones.

Family history

If your mother, father, sister, or brother has had osteoporosis, you also have a risk, and this risk rises if there has been a history of fractures.

Eating disorders

Anorexia Nervosa or bulimia increase risk of osteoporotic fractures in the low back and hips.

Low calcium intake

Milk, yogurt and cheese are high in calcium. Some food groups (cereals, orange juice) are fortified with calcium. If you avoid high calcium foods over a lifetime, you are at high risk for osteoporosis.

Tobacco

It has been shown that tobacco use enhances the development of weak bones.

Lack of exercise

A lifetime of physical activity and plentiful calcium in your diet will strengthen your bones. The opposite is true if you are sedentary.

Excess alcohol consumption

Men who drink too much alcohol are prone to osteoporosis because excess alcohol consumption reduces bone formation probably be interfering with the bodies ability to absorb calcium from the gastrointestinal tract.

Excess caffeinated soda consumption

Caffeine has a diuretic effect and may increase the loss of minerals such as calcium from the urine, plus it interferes with calcium absorption from the gastrointestinal tract.

Phosphoric acid in soda may change the acid-base balance in the blood and this, too, can contribute to bone loss.

You can somewhat negate these soda effects by increasing your intake of calcium and vitamin D either from supplements or dietary sources.

Depression

A major depression has been shown to increase bone loss.

Estrogen exposure

Estrogen helps prevent osteoporosis. If you had an early start of your menstrual periods coupled with a late menopause, you have been exposed to estrogen the longest possible time. Therefore you have less risk to develop osteoporosis. The reverse is true if you started your menstrual periods late and had an early menopause.

You are also put at greater risk if you had surgical removal of the ovaries before age forty-five without taking estrogen replacement therapy.

Medical illnesses and surgical procedures that prevent calcium absorption from the stomach

Surgical removal of the stomach puts you at greater risk.

You are at greater risk if you have the following medical conditions that impair your bodies ability to absorb calcium: Crohn's disease (an inflammatory bowel disease), hyperthyroidism (an overactive thyroid gland), Cushing's disease (an overactive adrenal gland), and anorexia nervosa (an eating disorder).

Cortisone medication

Anyone who has to take cortisone or cortisone-like medication long term is at risk for osteoporosis. Chronic cortisone use can cause bone loss. Bone density studies should be done to evaluate this possibility, and it may be necessary to take other medication to impede osteoporosis development.

Thyroid hormone

Too much thyroid hormone can promote bone loss. This can occur if your thyroid gland is overactive, or if it is underactive, and you take thyroid hormone replacement therapy in too large a dose.

Other medications

Certain diuretics can cause the kidneys to excrete more calcium thus possibly promoting osteoporosis.

Also heparin used to thin the blood, aluminum-based antacids, some medications taken to control seizures, and some chemotherapy agents used for breast cancer that block estrogen, can cause bone loss

Osteoporosis risk factor questions

Are you a woman?	__Yes __No
And are you past the menopause?	__Yes __No
Are you a man?	__Yes __No
And are you sixty-five years old or older?	__Yes __No
Are you Caucasian or from Southeast Asia?	__Yes __No
Are you a woman and do you weigh less than 127 pounds?	__Yes __No
Are you a slim small boned man?	__Yes __No
Has your mother, father, sister, or brother had osteoporosis?	__Yes __No

Have you been diagnosed with anorexia nervosa or bulimia?   __Yes __No

Do you rarely eat cheese, yogurt, milk, cereals and juices fortified with calcium?
    __Yes __No

Do you smoke?   __Yes __No

Do you exercise at least every other day for a half hour?   __Yes __No

Do you drink at least two alcoholic drinks per day?   __Yes __No

Do you frequently drink caffeinated soda drinks?   __Yes __No

Have you been treated for depression recently?   __Yes __No

Did you start your menstrual periods after age fourteen and did you stop them in your forties?   __Yes __No

Have you been diagnosed with any of the following: Hyperthyroidism, Cushing's disease, Anorexia Nervosa, or Crohn's disease?   __Yes __No

Have you taken cortisone medication for many months or years?   __Yes __No

Have you taken thyroid hormone for many months or years?   __Yes __No

Have you taken diuretics, anti-seizure medications, heparin, or chemotherapy agents for breast cancer?   __Yes __No

CHAPTER 16

DEPRESSION

Five to eight percent of the adult population suffers from major depression, a persistent illness that can significantly interfere with your life in terms of mental and physical problems. It is the major cause of disability in many countries including the United States.

Untreated depression can lead to suicide.

It affects women twice as much as men.

Besides major depression, also know as unipolar depression, there is a lesser form known as dysthymia (less severe than major depression, but chronic), and there is also bipolar depression, a combination of depression and mania (elevated mood, irritability, increased energy).

Usually the first bout of depression occurs between the ages of twenty and fifty.

Senior citizens are especially vulnerable, as are those who are experiencing great life-style changes.

Depression risk factors

Age

You are more susceptible if you are between the ages of twenty and fifty and if you are a senior citizen.

Marital state

Your risk for major depression greatly increases if you are unhappily married, separated, or divorced.

Prior episodes of depression

If you have been previously depressed, your chance for a repeat episode is somewhat greater.

Family history

Your risk is increased if members of your immediate family have suffered from major depression. The same holds true for manic depression.

Depression risk factor questions

Are you between the ages of twenty and fifty, or over age sixty-five?   __Yes __No

Are you unhappily married, separated, or divorced?   __Yes __No

Have you had a lengthy prior bout of depression?   __Yes __No

Has a parent, brother, or sister had severe depression?   __Yes __No

CHAPTER 17

ANXIETY

Excessive worry and anxiety, out of proportion to the situation, characterizes the clinical syndrome of anxiety. Worries about health, family, money, job, school, etcetera dominates thinking, so that one has difficulty functioning. Physical symptoms are common.

Anxiety risk factors

Stress

If you perceive a situation as stressful, it will be so.

A build up of stress will often cause anxiety that can interfere with your proper functioning and impact your life adversely.

Illness

You are more prone to anxiety if you suffer with a chronic illness.

Hormonal effect

Hyperthyroidism, hyperparathyroidism, Cushing's syndrome (overactive adrenal or pituitary glands), and diabetic hypoglycemia (low blood sugar), all result in increased hormonal activity that can cause anxiety.

Family history

A close family member who suffers from anxiety increases your risk for same.

Recent psychological or physical trauma

You are at increased risk for anxiety if you experience severe physical, sexual, or emotional abuse.

Excess sugar or chocolate

In some susceptible individuals, excess sugar and chocolate can trigger anxiety.

Medications

Anxiety can be caused by caffeine, diet pills, No Doze, cortisone and asthma medications.

Some central nervous depressants like alcohol, sleeping pills, tranquilizers and narcotics can cause anxiety once the medication is withdrawn.

Anxiety risk factor questions

Do you perceive that you are under extreme stress of late?   __Yes __No

Are you under a doctor's care for a chronic illness?   __Yes __No

Have you been treated for hyperthyroidism, hyperparathyroidism, Cushing's syndrome, diabetic hypoglycemia?   __Yes __No

Have you experienced severe physical, sexual, or emotional abuse?   __Yes __No

Are you in the habit of eating lots of sugar or chocolate?   __Yes __No

Do you use caffeine drinks, take diet pills or cortisone or asthma medication, or use No Doze to stay awake?   __Yes __No

Have you recently stopped taking central nervous depressants like alcohol, sleeping pills, tranquilizers, or narcotics?   __Yes __No

CHAPTER 18

DISCUSSION

That concludes the information and questions on risk factors. I hope you took the risk factor tests and understand the importance of being proactive in terms of your own health. Share these results with your personal physician.

What you've read to this point should have given you a clearer understanding about risk factors and their place in early detection and prevention of disease. These risk factors have evolved as research continues, and they will continue to evolve as we learn from ongoing research efforts, clinical experience, and genetic advances.

I am stressing again that you take your own risk factor analysis, because you will learn a great deal about yourself and your potential risks for specific illnesses. This will enable you to practice early detection and take preventive measures.

If you are a normal risk adult and do not have risk factors for a specific illness, then the U.S. Preventive Services Task Force recommends certain screening procedures to be performed at intervals. You can get this information from this website—www.ahrq.gov/clinic/uspstfix.htm.

The medical profession gathers a medical history from a patient one of three ways:

a) A physician or other healthcare worker asks questions directly of the patient;

b) The patient fills out a paper questionnaire;

c)   The patient is interviewed by a computer.

All these methods do not fully include a specific illness-oriented risk factor analysis, and I view that as a failing, so I am advocating that risk factors for those diseases that are the leading causes of morbidity and mortality be included in all new patient history gathering interactions and physical examinations—whatever form it takes (see appendix 1).

You are being urged to take charge of your own healthcare.

Again: If you are to learn about yourself and take charge of your health, you are going to have to be proactive, and if you are to be proactive you will need to do one of two things: Take the risk factor analysis; and get a complete medical examination.

Following this you will need to be thoroughly educated as to all your medical problems. And verbal education is not enough. You will need everything in writing. You will need a summary list—(see appendix 2), and it should be stored on your computer, or stored on the internet, or kept in a drawer or file cabinet, or preferably kept on your person (wallet) so that you will have instant access to it for all contingencies.

Physicians need your help. If we are to take care of as many patients as we do, we need you to be aware of your problems. Question us when you don't understand. Don't fail to get second, or third, or more opinions. Get and store copies of your medical records. Review them often. Stay educated—(see appendix 3).

The medical profession is depending on you.

APPENDIX 1

COMPLETE MEDICAL EXAMINATION

Part 1: The Medical History

> Biographical Data
>
> Chief Complaint
>
> Present Illness
>
> Past History
>
> Family History (at least three generational)
>
> Habits
>
> Social History
>
> System Review of all organ systems

Part 2: Risk factor analysis

Part 3: The Physical Examination

> General

Vital signs

Skin, Hair and Nails

Head

Eyes

Ears

Nose and Sinuses

Mouth and Throat

Lymphatic System

Cardiovascular

Pulmonary

Gastrointestinal

Genitourinary

Gynecological

Musculoskeletal

Neurological

Part 4: Laboratory data

Complete Blood Count

Urinalysis

Established screening blood chemistry tests—about thirty.

A new series of blood tests—(250 biological markers known as Biophysical 250)—is currently being made available, and may allow the very early detection of some diseases before they become clinically obvious—a boon for early detection.

Part 5: Medical report and Summary list

APPENDIX 2

SUMMARY LIST

1. Established significant medical diagnosis of a chronic nature that must be followed long term and is vital to current and future decision making. For example, diabetes mellitus, congestive heart failure, hypertension, Crohn's disease, osteoarthritis, multiple sclerosis, manic depressive disorder.

2. Allergies to drugs, and the type of allergic reaction.

3. Known significant surgical or invasive procedures that have been performed. For example, quadruple coronary artery bypass graft, hip replacement, cholecystectomy (gall bladder removal), total abdominal hysterectomy (removal of uterus, fallopian tubes, ovaries), breast biopsy, appendectomy. Listing an old appendectomy is important if, in the future, your physician will have to make a diagnosis as to the cause of lower abdominal pain.

4. Important symptoms should be listed by your doctor if he has not yet established a reason for the symptom. Once the symptom is explained, the diagnosis can displace the symptom. For example: left arm pain subsequently discovered to be due to coronary artery disease.

5. A social risk factor that may be impacting your health. For example: a bitter divorce.

6. Medication list (name and dose) including complementary medications (herbs), vitamins, prescription medications and over the counter medications taken on a regular basis.

7. Immunizations

An example of a medical summary list:

1. Status post quadruple artery bypass graft (anterior descending branch, right, two diagonal branches) 1996

2. Post cardiotomy syndrome—resolved

3. Allergy: anemia secondary to cardura and hytrin (resolved when medications discontinued)

4. Elevated total cholesterol and reduced HDL cholesterol (resolved with therapy)

5. Premature atrial contractions

6. Hypertension

7. Benign prostatic hypertrophy (prostate cancer biopsy negative—2007)

8. Right inguinal herniorrhaphy 1998

9. Cataract surgery (right) 2005 (left) 2006

10. Immunizations Flu yearly—Pneumovacc 1995—DT 1998

Medications:

Toprol 100 mgm—one every morning

Hydrochlorothiazide 25 mgm—one every morning

Saw palmetto 320 mgm—one every morning

Finasteride 5 mgm—one every morning

Centrum Silver multivitamin—one every morning

Omega 3 fatty acids 1000 mgm—one every morning and evening

Flo max 0.4 mgm—two every evening

Lisinopril 20 mgm—two every evening

Simvastatin 20 mgm—one every evening

Halfprim (aspirin) 162 mgm—one every evening

Another example of a medical summary list:

1. Atrial fibrillation

2. Hypertension

3. Degenerative arthritis both knees

4. Endometrial hyperplasia (resolved—see problem 5)

5. Total abdominal hysterectomy 1994

6. Allergies—NONE

7. Immunizations Flu yearly—Pneumovacc 1998—DT 2000

Medication:

Norvasc 5 mgm every morning

Furosemide 20 mgm every morning

Atacand 32 mgm every morning

Ziac 5/6.25 every morning

Warfarin Sodium 4mgm every evening except 2 mgm Tue and Thur

APPENDIX 3

"Knowledge is of two kinds. We know a subject ourselves, or we know where we can find information upon it."

Samuel Johnson

(1709–1784)

WEB SITES FOR PATIENTS

GOOGLE: Google is not a specific medical web site, but since it has information on anything it can be used as one. A click—and the world's knowledge is at your fingertips. If you are seeking medical information, you can get it on Google. If you are seeking a medical organization and don't know the web site address, type the name of the organization and Google will direct you. I have done this many times.

ALLREFER.COM

Includes extensive information on alternative medicine, diet and nutrition, health news, injuries and wounds, surgery and procedures, symptoms guide, special topics, tests and exams, pictures and images, medical encyclopedia. In addition there are non-medical topics.

CANCER.GOV

This is the web-site for the National Cancer Institute. Every form of cancer is discussed. The most up-to-date information is available and includes: treatment, prevention, genetics, cause, clinical trials, cancer literature, research and related information, screening and testing and statistics.

CENTER FOR DISEASE CONTROL AND PREVENTION (CDC)

Comprehensive information about birth defects, disabilities, diseases and conditions, emergency preparedness and response, environmental health, genetics and genomics, health promotion, injury and violence, travelers health, vaccines and immunizations, workplace safety and health. There are books and journals listed as well as national and state statistics and growth charts.

FAMILYDOCTOR.ORG

Discussion on all conditions from A to Z. Information on healthy living, smart patient guide, women, men, seniors, parents and kids, over the counter guide, health tools. If you are looking for a family physician, type in a zip code, click, and they will be identified.

HEALTHFINDER U.S. DEPARTMENT OF HEALTH AND HUMAN SERVICES

Diseases, conditions and injuries from A to Z, drug database, online checkups, consumer guide, find a provider, find a facility, health news, clinical trials update, weekly health newsletter.

HIV INSITE, UNIVERSITY OF SAN FRANSISCO SCHOOL OF MEDICINE CHI CENTER FOR HIV ONFORMATION

This website provides a comprehensive knowledge base on the latest medical information on HIV, latest research information and preventive measures.

MAYOCLINIC.COM

They have developed a very complete web site that discusses many diseases and conditions. These are written by Mayo Clinic physicians whose picture accompanies the article. They also have information on drugs and supplements, treatment decisions, health living for all ages, health tools including calculators, self assessment tools, quizzes, slide shows, videos and an ask the specialist feature enabling anyone to query one of the Mayo physicians. This web site is my personal favorite that is geared to patients.

MEDLINEPLUS A SERVICE OF THE U.S. NATIONAL LIBRARY OF MEDICINE AND THE NATIONAL INSTITUTE OF HEALTH

Health topics on diseases, conditions and wellness, information on drugs and supplements, medical encyclopedia with pictures and diagrams, medical dictionary, current health news, directory for doctors, dentists and hospitals, local health services, libraries and organizations.

NOAH NEW YORK ONLINE ACCESS TO HEALTH

Disorders and conditions by body locations/systems, local health resources, groups, procedures and medicine, health and wellness, health index from A to Z and page of the month.

WEBMD.COM

They have condition centers with comprehensive information on diseases. There is also information on drugs and herbs, medical library, health tools, find a doctor, clinical trials health plans and more, women, men, life style, pregnancy and family, diet and nutrition, chats and boards.

www.ahrq.gov/clinic/uspstfix.htm

Try the above:

From the US Preventive Services Task Force. They provide recommendations for screening services for EVERY ILLNESS YOU CAN THINK OF! Kept current and up to date.

An independent panel of experts in primary care and prevention systematically reviews the evidence of effectiveness and develops recommendations for clinical preventive services.

BOOKS ON MEDICAL SUBJECTS FOR PATIENTS

JOHNS HOPKIN'S FAMILY HEALTH BOOK

This is an excellent book for patients. It is very comprehensive and includes:

1. Staying healthy: eating well, staying active, staying fit, everyday safety, smoking and how to stop.

2. Healthcare over the life course: family history, genetics and your health, pregnancy and childbirth, infancy, pre-school, teen years, adulthood, senior years.

3. First aid and emergency care

4. Body systems and disorders: an excellent discussion of all body organ systems.

5. Becoming a partner in your healthcare: taking charge of your healthcare, preparing for surgery, how to use medications, home care and long-term care, death and dying.

6. Appendices: medication directory, glossary, growth charts, living wills and advanced directives, measurement conversions, laboratory tests.

7. Color atlas of anatomy, disorders and diseases.

MAYO CLINIC FAMILY HEALTH BOOK

Also an excellent book and it includes:

1. Living well: nutrition, fitness, stress management, other.

2. Common conditions and concerns through life's stages: growth and deveplo-ment, health issues common to children and adults, death and dying.

3. Making sense of your symptoms.

4. First aid and emergency care.

5. Diseases and disorders: signs and symptoms, description of condition, how diagnosed, treatment options.

6. Tests and treatments: tests, medications, surgery, pain management, comple-mentary and alternative therapies.

MERCK MANUAL OF MEDICAL INFORMATION 2ND HOME EDITION

1. Fundamentals.

2. Drugs.

3. Disorders of all organ systems.

THE LIFETIME HEALTH JOURNAL by Karolina Kowiaki

This book will teach you how to keep records of your healthcare throughout your life. This is a critically important issue that will allow you to be able to be an active participant in your healthcare.

1. Introduction.

2. Childhood health record.

3. Adult and long term health record.

NOTHING ABOUT ME WITHOUT ME: A PRACTICAL GUIDE FOR AVOIDING MEDICAL ERRORS by Melinda Ashton M.D. & Linda Richards R.N. MBA

This book is an excellent summary of how to avoid medical errors. There is a patient example illustrating each point.

1. Exploring the issue: aspects of hospital care, patient testing.

2. The many facets of hospital care.

3. Managing medications.

4. Visit to the doctor's office

5. When more than one doctor is involved.

6. Choosing a doctor to satisfy you.

7. When children need medical care.

8. Final thoughts.

HOW TO SAVE YOUR OWN LIFE. THE EIGHT STEPS ONLY YOU CAN TAKE TO MANAGE AND CONTROL YOUR HEALTHCARE by Maria Saved M.D.

1. Trusting yourself as the real expert about your health.

2. Collecting and studying copies of your medical records.

3. Researching your conditions, disease and injuries.

4. Learning which immunizations, exams, and tests you need and when.

5. Helping your doctor help you.

6. Participating in decisions about your treatment options.

7. Knowing how to get the best care in the hospital.

8. Find the courage to treat yourself right.

9. Epilogue: here's to your health.

10. Appendix: copies of actual medical records.

YOU THE SMART PATIENT AN INSIDER'S HANDBOOK TO GETTING THE RIGHT TREATMENT BY Michael F. Roizen M.D. & Mehmet C. Oz M.D.

This book tells readers how to take charge of their own healthcare. The book is written with the collaboration of the Joint Commission, the accrediting organization for all healthcare organizations.

The End

978-0-595-46739-6
0-595-46739-3